Yoga Essentials 101

A Beginner's Handbook to the Practice of Yoga

By Essence McDaniels

Table of Contents

Chapter 1: Beginning With the Yogic Tree

Yoga unlocks something deep within you. While fitness studios and gyms boast of the physical benefits of yoga, this ancient practice is far more than just another workout. Yoga has the power to unlock something deep within the human mind and allows us to access the true nature of ourselves.

This practice was designed to work in harmony with the human body and utilizes anatomical principles that modern science has only recently started to understand. These ancient teachings were created through enlightened observations of all types of life. Within our practice, we work to become harmonious with the world around us, focus our mind and open our senses. We learn how to discern between the things that we cannot change (isvara pranidhana) and the things that we can actually change (tapah).

Ancient yogis believed that human beings had three bodies: the physical, causal and astral. According to their viewpoint, yoga was intended to move between the layers of these three bodies. From the start of your first yoga class, you begin to integrate the mind, body and breath. With practice, you can go beyond the basic limitations of your physical form to unlock the true potential of yoga.

What Is Yoga?

The word yoga is from a Sanskrit word, yuj, that means to bind or yoke. This word can be used to mean union or to concentrate one's attention. In essence, yoga means the yoking of all the powers of your soul, mind and body to God. It is a way of developing a disciplined intellect and controlled emotions. Traditionally, it is considered to be one of the six mainstays of Indian philosophy. Originally, this ancient practice was codified and standardized in the Yoga Sutras by Patanjali.

It is unknown when Sri Patanjali lived, and some historians are uncertain if a single person actually wrote the Yoga Sutras. Currently, historians believe that the sutras were written between 5,000 B.C. and 300 A.D. Whether Patanjali actually wrote the sutras or not, historians know that he did not invent yoga. His main contribution was to write down and systematize the practices that already existed. Over the next 2,000 years, his sutras became the basis for all of the yoga and meditation styles that developed.

In Indian philosophy, all of the world is permeated by the Supreme Universal Spirit.

Each human soul is just a small part of this entire spirit. Through yoga, Indian tradition says that each person can unify and commune with the universal spirit. Someone who follows this path is known as a yogin or yogi. In many ways, yoga is like meditation. Meditation can be used to break the cycle of samsara and suffering. Likewise, yoga can be used to free yourself of the pains and sorrows of normal existence.

The body is our chief instrument for acting our every desire, thought and will. While you use your body in daily life, it is undisciplined and uncontrolled. Your mind follows your body's tendency to be undisciplined. If you use yoga to discipline your body, you can also discipline your mind. By using yoga to discipline the body, we can bring the mind and emotions under control. Each asana is perfected through practice, so it in essence becomes a spiritual mudra. A mudra means a seal, and a seal was used in ancient times to confirm the sender of the message.

In a way, the human body is also a seal. We have to unlock what lies behind our own seal by learning what the body conveys. We are a closed book that contains frustrations, aches and emotional agony that we are not aware of. In the Eastern tradition, you are a discoverer and an adventurer who investigates your mind, soul and body. By performing yoga, you unlock the seals that prevent you from learning the true nature of your awareness. Yoga encourages intuitive perception and encourages reflection. As such, it goes beyond the physical to activate all types of human awareness. You start by training the central nervous systems and your body, but you end up developing self-mastery. Before long, you begin to gain control of your mind, speech and emotions.

The Eight Stages of Yoga

In Patanjali's Yoga Sutra, he discusses the eight limbs of yoga. In essence, yoga is like a tree with many limbs. To truly master the art of yoga, you must master each of the eight limbs. These limbs are yama (universal moral commandments), niyama (self-purification by discipline), asana (posture), pranayama (rhythmic control of the breath), pratyahara (freeing the mind from the senses and exterior factors), dharana (concentration), dhyana (meditation) and samadhi (a level of super-consciousness developed through exceptional meditation that allows you to become unified with the universal spirit).

Each component of yoga has a separate identity, but it is a part of the same tree. To truly practice yoga, you must combine all of these eight stages and practice regularly. Through these stages, you can deepen your knowledge of the self and your consciousness. From the mind (manas), you go through a process that is similar to the unraveling of an onion. As you progress, you go through the intellect (buddhi), the will (samkalpa), discriminating consciousness (prajna or viveka-khyati), conscience (sad-asad-viveka) and the self (atma).

Yama

Yama is the collective commandments that are universal across time and place. These include the great vows of truth, non-stealing, non-violence, continence and non-covetousness. If these seem similar to Christianity's Ten Commandments, there is a reason for that. Over thousands of years, philosophers, yogis and saints have realized the underlying moral commandments that underlie human existence. These great vows are similar across religions because their basis is universal.

When you can abandon hatred and embrace non-violence, all that remains is an all-embracing love. The yogi learns to be truthful with himself and only says, thinks or does things that he believes are true. He or she is capable of controlling their thoughts and emotions. Continence allows you to see the divinity in everyone without facing sexual desire. In a similar fashion, yogis are able to avoid coveting others items, feeling jealous, acting with violence or stealing because they recognize that desire only furthers the cycle of suffering.

Niyama

This stage is translated as self-purification and is made up of purity, austerity, scripture study, contentment and surrendering to a higher power. When practicing niyama, the yogi recognizes that he is subject to the desires of the body and mind. To maintain purity, he keeps himself and his surroundings clean. Spiritually, the yogi works to root out the six evils of anger, pride, passion, greed, malice and infatuation. By removing these destructive thoughts and feelings, he is able to fill his mind with constructive thoughts that encourage him on the path to divinity.

Being content means that you are able to control your desires, feel cheerful and have a balanced mind. Meanwhile, austerity allows you to discipline your body in a way that lets it persevere through hardship. As a result, of study and austerity, you can focus your attention on searching for the truth and becoming self-realized. When these skills are learned, you are able to surrender yourself to the world and allow fate to take control. The virtues of niyama are necessary for calming disturbed minds and ensuring peace.

Asanas

The most well-known aspect of yoga is the asanas. These are known in English as the postures. In your body, you have three humors (doshas) known as the phlegm (kapha), bile (pitta) and wind (vata). When these humors are in balance, you enjoy good health and strong digestion. Life is a combination of perception, the body, action, mind, ego, soul and intellect. The mind bridges the body and soul, but it needs help to remain in balance. Through regular practice, asanas help to balance out the humors and enhance the connection between all parts of your mind and soul.

Pranayama

Pranayama is a conscious way of prolonging your inhales, exhales and retention of air. When you inhale, you are bringing in primeval energy through the breath. As you hold this breath, you are savoring the energy. Each exhale allows you to send out the thoughts and emotions from your mind. As you empty your lungs, you are emptying yourself of the preconceived notions that are holding you back. In essence, you are surrendering your individual energy for the primeval energy.

Constant practice of pranayama helps to encourage a strong will power, healthy mind and sound judgment. Together, pranayama and pratyahara are known as the inner quests. They help you to regulate your breathing so that you can control your mind. With time, you can free your senses from the enslavement of desire.

Pratyahara

Pratyahara refers to the discipline that allows you to bring your senses, emotions and mind under control. In a way, it plays a dual role. While it seeks to satisfy your senses, pratyahara also works to unite one with the self. It quiets the senses enough that you can turn your focus inward and meet with the divine. Pratyahara is the withdrawal of the senses and emancipation of the mind.

Dharana and Dhyana

Dharana sounds simple, but few things in yoga are really as straightforward as they seem. This practice is the concentration on a single point. It could also be used as total attention on what you are doing without ruffling the mind. With dharana, you encourage an inner awareness that allows you to integrate your intelligence while releasing all tension. When it is continued for an extended period of time, it is considered dhyana (meditation). For Westerners, dharana and dhyana are recognized in practices like mindfulness meditation.

Samadhi

When you are able to maintain the state of dhyana for a long time without interruptions, you can merge into samadhi. In this state, you lose all sense of your individual identity as you merge with the object of your meditation. During samadhi, the sadhaka loses their consciousness of their body, mind, intelligence, breath and ego. They are at a state of being where infinite wisdom, humility, simplicity and purity take precedence. Someone in this state can be said to have achieved enlightenment. To anyone who approaches, the sadhaka shines enlightenment and truth.

The yoga of action or karma yoga includes the stages of yama, asana and niyama. These stages are designed to keep the mind and body pure. Meanwhile, pranayama, dharana and pratyahara are part of the yoga of knowledge (jnana). In these stages, you gain knowledge as you seek the universal truth. In the last two stages of dhyana and samadhi, you merge your mind, intelligence and body to become the Self. These last stages are known as the yoga of love and devotion (bhakti). Karma, bhakti and jnana yoga all flow together to form the pathway that allows you to move toward beatitude and true freedom.

Chapter 2: Dynamic Breathing: Nourishing for the Body and Soul

Cells are the basic building block of human life, and the human body has about 100 trillion cells. Each cell includes a cytoplasm, cell membrane and nucleus. The membrane keeps the cell safe from the external environment, while allowing nutrients to penetrate the membrane. These nutrients are then used to fuel the cell's functions in life. Like any metabolic activity, waste is produced in the process. The waste is removed through the same cell membrane that allows nutrients to flow inwards.

When waste cannot leave or nutrients cannot come in, the cell dies from toxicity or starvation. Yoga functions around the same concepts as the cell. Prana and apana refer to the concepts of nourishing life and removing waste.

Prana and Apana

In Sanskrit, pra- is a prefix that means before, and "an" is a verb that means to live, breathe or blow. As a result, prana means to nourish a living thing and bring nourishment inward. When it is capitalized, Prana also refers to the universal term that refers to the creative life force.

Since every living being needs to bring in nourishment and excrete waste, apana is a necessary counterbalance to prana. "Apa" means off or down, so apana refers to eliminating waste or the waste that is eliminated.

In the cell, the membrane must be in a perfect balance to allow nutrients to flow through and waste to flow outward. If the membrane is too permeable, the cell loses its integrity and can implode. A cell that is not permeable enough starves without waste flowing outward and fresh nutrients flowing inward. All living things use the same principles.

These polarities are represented through sthira and sukha. Sthira means solid, strong, permanent or nonfluctuating in Sanskrit. Meanwhile, sukha means easy, pleasant or mild. It can also mean the state of being free of obstacles. Every living being is a balance of these two states. Like a suspension bridge must be strong yet flexible, the human body must have a balance of strength and flexibility.

Sukha also means good (su) and space (kha). This implies that your body must have an empty space at its center to function as an axle. As long as you have good space at your center, you are able to create functional connections between the rest of your being.

The Body's Pathways for Nutrition and Waste

The human body is designed with pathways for nutrients and waste. While these pathways are more complex than a cell membrane, they are still fairly easy to understand in terms of apana and prana. In the digestion system, the human body is open at the top and bottom. For your body, prana is consumed in the form of food and drink. It is consumed at the top of your body through the top. As the solids and liquids move through the digestive processes, the nutrients are removed and waste is produced. At the bottom of the digestive system, the force of apana pushes solid and liquid waste from the body.

Prana is also brought into our bodies through the breath. The human body requires air to live as well as solid and liquid nourishment. In this form, it enters the lungs using the diaphragm and is exchanged in the capillaries and alveoli. Later, the waste gas is expelled through the same system. Prana brings air into the body, and apana expels it through the body.

When a fetus is in the mother's womb, the mother is responsible for breathing. Her lungs bring in the oxygen that is brought through the placenta and uterus to the umbilical cord. From there, oxygenated blood enters through the inferior vena cava and the liver. Both sides of the heart are connected so that the oxygen bypasses the lungs until the child is born. Fetal circulation is far different from the way people breathe after birth.

Once you are born, you are severed from the umbilical cord that links you to your mother. For the first time, you had to breathe in air in order to survive. This first breath is the most important and forceful breath that you have ever taken. The moment it happens, it causes massive changes to the circulatory system. Blood pumps into both sides of the lungs, and special vessels shut down the fetal circulation. Ligaments develop to support the abdominal organs.

This first breath is so forceful because it has to overcome inactive lung tissue and create tension. It is three to four times stronger than a normal breath. At the same time, the fetus suddenly leaves a supportive, fluid-filled environment and is forced to support itself in gravity.

Babies are typically supported and swaddled in the early months, so it may seem like mobility and stability are not important. In reality, infants begin to learn posture and complex skills like breathing from the moment they are born. The immense strength and skill it takes for an infant to lift its head is impressive. The head takes up a quarter of the infant's body length, so it requires many muscles to bear the weight. For the next year, the infant continues to experience postural development as it learns to sit, crawl and walk. The lumbar curve develops as the infant learns to walk and finishes developing when you are about 10 years old.

To live on earth, your body must integrate breath, posture, sukha, sthira, prana and apana. If any of these functions are out of balance, the other bodily functions suffer. With this viewpoint, yoga is a way to make sure that the body's systems are integrated so that you spend more time in sukha than in dukha.

You Don't Breathe: The Universe Breathes You

You breathe constantly, so it is easy to take this skill for granted. The process of moving air in and out of your lungs is what shapes your bodily cavities. There are essentially two cavities related to breathing: the abdominal and thoracic cavities. The abdominal cavity contains the large intestines, stomach, small intestines, bladder, spleen, liver, gall bladder, pancreas and kidneys. In the thoracic cavity, we find the heart and lungs. Both of these cavities are open on one side. While the thoracic cavity opens at the top, the abdominal cavity opens at the body.

Between the two cavities, the diaphragm forms a shared barrier. The cavities are both supported by the spine and change shape. While they both change shape with each breath, the way that they change shape is different.

The abdominal cavity could be compared to a water balloon. When you squeeze one side of a water balloon, the other side bulges out. It is impossible to compress water, so one side must bulge when another is compressed. When you breath, your abdominal cavity performs the same type of compression. The shape may change, but the volume remains the same. If you drink or eat excessively, you increase the volume in the abdominal cavity by filling your stomach, bladder and intestines. Whenever the abdominal cavity increases in volume, it causes the thoracic cavity to decrease. This is the reason why it is harder to breathe after a large meal or when you are pregnant.

Unlike the abdominal cavity, the thoracic cavity will change in shape and in volume. It is essentially a gas-filled container like an accordion or a normal balloon. When you pull on an accordion, you increase the volume inside as air is pulled in. When you push the sides of the accordion together, it causes the air to be pushed out and the volume decreases. The thoracic cavity does the same action.

Imagine that you have an accordion placed on a water balloon inside of you. Every time you breathe, the accordion expands and pushes into the water balloon. This forces the abdominal cavity (the water balloon) to change shape, although the volume remains the same. When you exhale, the accordion shrinks and the water balloon is able to expand again. If you have effective breathing, your body's cavities are easily able to change shape to accommodate the expansion of the thoracic cavity.

Volume and pressure are intrinsically related. When volume increases, pressure decreases. When volume drops, pressure rises. Air will always move to areas that have lower pressure. This means that decreasing the pressure in the thoracic cavity will cause the air to flow inside.

You do not pull air into your body. It is easy to mistake breathing for something that you force to happen. In reality, you do not breathe; the universe breathes you. Atmospheric pressure on earth is at about 14.7 pounds per square inch. This pressure is always around you and never changes. Since air naturally flows from areas of higher pressure to lower pressure, the only reason you can breathe is because your diaphragm lowers the pressure in your chest as it expands. This decreased pressure is what causes the air to flow into your lungs through a process known as passive recoil.

For the universe to breathe you, your body's cavities must be able to change shape. This is done primarily through a single muscle known as the diaphragm. The diaphragm is like a parachute or jellyfish in shape. This muscle is connected through supportive tendons to organs in the body that allow it to retain its shape.

The lower fibers of the diaphragm are attached through flexible cartilage and ligaments. Meanwhile, the upper fibers are attached to the heart. The central tendon that connects to the heart is actually developed when humans are just in the embryonic stage of development. Because of these anchors, the diaphragm can be used to lift the rib cage up or to expand the stomach. While both forms of breath are caused by the diaphragm, it is healthier for the body to expand the stomach. Both types of breath use the diaphragm, but only belly breathing uses the diaphragm efficiently. If you can learn through yoga to breathe with your stomach instead of your rib cage, you can get the highest level of efficiency from your breath.

Yoga asanas and pranayama (breathing practice) are designed to teach your body how to use accessory muscles to change the shape of your cavities and utilize belly breathing to intake air. All of the accessory muscles must be activated and strengthened to encourage stable, efficient breathing.

While we have only focused on one type of diaphragm, there are actually three diaphragms: pelvic, vocal and respiratory. In ujjayi, yoga coordinates all of the diaphragms to protect the spine. During ujjayi breathing, a back pressure is created in the body's cavities that provides a protective support for the spine. This can occur during salutations or extension movements. By coordinating the diaphragms (bandhas), you can create better stability in your body. One of the reasons why you instinctively hold your breath during some movements is because your body wants to protect itself from energy. If you can master ujjayi breathing, your body does not need this instinctive response to be protected.

Diet, Posture and Techniques for Pranayama

Food is an anatomical requirement for humans to live, and you would not be able to practice yoga without it. The body must receive food that contains the right blend of vitamins, carbohydrates, proteins, minerals and fats to be healthy. In yoga and pranayama, it is recommended that you balance your food intake according to three types:

Sattvic: This type of food promotes happiness, health and longevity.

Rajasic: This food classification produces excitement and can cause the consciousness to become dull.

Tamasic: This type of food causes disease and can impede spiritual progress.

While the state of the mind determines your yogic potential greatly, the food you eat can influence your success. Sattvic, vegetarian food will help to produce a clear and unwavering mind that is ideal for pranayama. Yoga texts recommend eating only when saliva flows and you are hungry. Otherwise, your body is not able to absorb the nutrients in the food. Ancient texts also recommend filling your stomach three-quarters with food, one-quarter with fluids and one-quarter with breath. This recommendation is also mirrored in other societies. In Japan, for instance, traditional proverbs recommend eating until you are three-quarters full.

Fasting is not necessary for most yogis. Your body must be nourished to function at its best, and fasting removes this nourishment. Moderate food intake helps you to maintain your alertness, strength and vigor. When you are doing asanas, make sure to do them on an empty stomach. If this is not possible for you, wait at least an hour after a light meal and four hours after a heavy meal. You can eat after your asanas once 30 minutes have passed.

If you are having bowel problems, upside-down poses will generally help to encourage movement. Otherwise, you should make sure that your bowels and bladder are empty before doing asanas. You should never attempt advanced asanas without emptying your bowels first.

For pranayama practice, you should wait at least six hours after a meal before practicing. If this is difficult, you can drink a cup of tea, milk or cocoa to satiate your body.

Choosing the Time and Place

According to the Hatha Yoga Pradipika, pranayama should be practiced at least four times a day. Ideally, you should practice in the early morning, at noon, evening and at midnight. If this is not possible, you should set a goal of at least 15 minutes a day. Consistency in your pranayama practice is important for you to make progress in a healthy, stable and efficient manner.

For asanas, the best time to practice is in the early morning or late in the evening. While morning practice will help you to wake up in the morning, evening practice removes the fatigue of the day and leaves you feeling calm. You should avoid practicing after being in the hot sun for too long, and you should choose a clean location. Whenever possible, pick a spot that is free from loud noises or insects. A mat or folded blanket should be placed on the floor to give you a safe place to do your asanas.

Watch Your Physical Posture

During pranayama, you should sit in a way that does not cause undue strain on any part of your body. Your tongue should remain passive or saliva will begin to accumulate. If this happens, swallow right before you exhale, but after you have held your breath.

Sitting is the most comfortable and effective way to do pranayama. A folded blanket, meditation pillow or another pillow can help you to maintain your posture comfortably. As you are sitting, you will want to make sure that your back is erect from the spine to the neck and perpendicular to the floor. This may be painful at first as your body develops the necessary muscles to support itself, but it will become more comfortable over time.

Each style of pranayama and meditative practice may recommend a different posture, so be aware that there are variations. While some practices allow your eyes to remain focused, it is often better to keep your eyes closed when you are just starting out. Closed eyes will keep outside actions or objects from distracting you.

Try to work toward an even ratio of inhales to exhales. If you inhale for five seconds, try to make sure that your exhales are also for five seconds. Even, steady breathing helps to encourage healthy nerves and a balanced temper. You should never do pranayama when you are too exhausted because your muscles would be too tired to stay erect. Be safe and listen to your body as you work toward a regular pranayama practice.

Chapter 3: Spinal Health and Happiness Through Yoga

Over millions of years, the spinal cord gradually developed and was an essential aspect of humanity's survival. As it developed, it became essential for life forms to move around and actively seek out nutrients. The skeletal spine was vital for delicate organs to be protected and nutrients to move through the body.

For animals to walk on two legs, a straight spine had to be created that balanced out gravity's destabilizing force on the body. This development allowed terrestrial creatures to raise up on two limbs and respond effectively to gravitational stress. Without a straightened spine, gravitational forces would have harmed the unsupported middle. The front-back curve of the spine was the first to emerge. Before long, the neck started to develop. Breathing structures began to move down in early creatures so that breathing apparatus and mobility could be ensured. This highly mobile structure allowed the neck to be turned precisely for quick looks around the environment. As a result, creatures with the ability had a survival advantage.

The human spine is unique among all animals because it included thoracic, sacral, cervical and lumbar curves. Only a biped requires both of these curves because these curves are essentially for you to walk and stand upright. Animals that do not stand upright do not need these two spinal cords to support their body against gravity. Our primate cousins only required a minimal cervical curve and no lumbar curve, which is why they are not considered to be a true biped. Our bodies' spines allow us to bear weight and move in the lower body. In the upper body, the spine allows us to reach items, grasp things and breathe.

Since we are descended from other animals, a fetus develops traits that resemble our ancestors like gills and a tail. These traits are quickly discarded once they develop since humans no longer need them. The first time our spine moves out of the primary curve of the fetal stage is at birth. As our heads navigate the curve of the birth canal, our necks go through the Iordotic curve for the first time ever. This causes the spine to immediately change shape and adopt its first real curve.

Over months and years, the spine develops as we grow. The cervical curve continues to develop when we hold our heads up at about three months, and it finishes forming when we sit upright at about nine months. When babies begin to walk instead of crawl at 12 to 18 months, the lumbar spine straightens out. At the age of three, the lumbar spine becomes concave. By the age of six, this concave shape is more readily visible. Once we reach the age of 10, the lumbar spine is fully developed.

From an engineering perspective, human beings have the highest center of gravity, the smallest support base and the heaviest head proportional to our weight of any animal. As a result, we are the world's least stable animal mechanically. Fortunately, yoga can help our bodies learn the intrinsic equilibrium, balance and flexibility that allow our spines to function effectively.

The Inner Workings of the Spine

The spinal column in our bodies has been designed to balance the compressive and tensile forces which we experience from movement and gravity. There are a total of 24 vertebrae that are bound together through capsular joints, discs and ligaments. They alternate between bones and soft tissue for a balance of active and passive elements. The passive elements (sthira) are the vertebrae. The active elements (sukha) in the spine are the facet joints, ligaments and intervertebral discs. Altogether, the passive and active elements function for an integrated system and stable equilibrium.

The Types of Spinal Movement

There are essentially four types of movements for the spine. The spine can do axial rotation, flexion, lateral flexion and extension. These four movements occur spontaneously throughout daily life without you ever having to think about it. Whether you are tying your shoes or reaching for a bag in the back seat, you are using your spine.

While you may do all of these movements naturally, yoga postures are designed to emphasize these movements. As you age, your spinal health is key to your life expectancy, ease of movement and general mobility. By practicing all four types of spinal movement through yoga, you can ensure the optimal spinal health.

In the following column, we have written out the degrees of motion that can be attained with each movement of your spine. While some individuals are more or less flexible than others, this range of motion is generally true for most people.

	Extension	Flexion	Total
Lumbar	35°	60°	95°
Thoracic	25°	45°	70°
Cervical	75°	40°	115°
Total	135°	145°	280°

In reality, a fifth range of motion actually exists for the spine. Known as an axial extension, this range of motion never happens spontaneously in day-to-day life. It is only occurs during "unnatural" situations like asanas.

The most simple movements of the spine are centered around the flexion curve. This primary curve occurs in the thoracic spine, and it is the same curve that you see when the fetus is in the womb. Thus, it is unsurprising that one of the most popular yoga poses that emphasizes this curve, child's pose, was named that way. Child's pose reflects the original curve of the spine, and many poses like corpse pose use the same shape. In corpse pose (savasana), the majority of the body is in contact with the floor. All of the secondary curves like the lumbar and cervical spine are actually off of the floor.

With this in mind, we can define spinal flexion as the increase in primary spinal curves and the decrease in secondary curves. The relationship between these two types of curves in the body is essentially reciprocal: the more you flex of one curve, the less the other will curve.

One of the best ways to see this curve in action is to use the cat and cow asanas. With your spine supported by the arms and thighs, it can produce flexion and extension shape changes. While your instructor normally tells you to inhale and exhale to cause the shape change, it is really the shape change that causes the inhalation and exhalation. When you do a spinal extension, it causes your breathing cavities to open up and inhale. Likewise, flexion forces you to exhale.

While it is often the case, spinal flexion is not the same thing as bending forward, and spinal extension is not the same thing as bending backward. Flexion and extension are only meant to refer to the relationship between one spinal curve and another. It is important as you learn yoga that you can start to recognize and copy the different types of spinal movement.

When we look at yoga poses that use twisting and lateral movements, it is important to consider the difference between spatial and spinal perspectives. Triangle pose is often discussed as a lateral stretch in yoga, and it is true that it lengthens the connective tissue that runs across the side of the body. At the same time, it is possible to lengthen the lateral line of the body without doing any noticeable lateral flexion of the spine. In triangle pose, a more lateral line could be made by spacing the feet wider and initiating all of the movement from the pelvis. This would also help to open up the hips.

Lateral flexion of the spine could also be encouraged by placing the feet closer together. This would provide increased stabilization between the thighs and pelvis, and it would also require more movement from the spine.

The fifth spinal movement, axial extension, is the simultaneous decrease in both the primary and secondary curves of the spine. As a result of this, the length of the spine is increased. Since the primary and secondary curves form a reciprocal relationship, axial extension is an "unnatural" movement. This means that an axial extension does not happen naturally unless you are making a conscious effort to attain it.

When you do an axial extension, it shifts the orientation of your breathing structures (bandhas). The pelvic, vocal and respiratory diaphragms become more stable. Meanwhile, the thoracic and abdominal cavities become limited.

As a result, your spinal length increases, but your breathing capacity decreases. This state is referred to as mahamudra in yoga, which translates as the great seal. Mahamudra can be done in supine, arm support, seated and standing positions. If you can achieve mahamudra during your yoga practice, it represents a supreme accomplishment because it shows that you are completely able to merge pranayama and asana practice.

Maintaining an Equilibrium Between Your Spine, Pelvis and Rib Cage

Even if all of the muscles attached to your spine would remove, your spine would not collapse. It is in a state of intrinsic equilibrium, so your spine is self-supporting. This same type of arrangement is found in both the pelvis and the rib cage. Bound together through mechanical tension, they are in a state of intrinsic equilibrium.

Yoga is able to achieve an exceptional impact on your body because it removes the obstructions and forces that prevent your body from changing. It builds a deep level of core support that allows your body to maintain its balance, stability and intrinsic equilibrium. This support does not depend solely on muscular effort because it is developed from the ways your ligaments, bone and cartilage interact. When these supports are activated alone, it is always because the extra muscular effort normally used is no longer needed.

It takes an exceptional amount of energy to exert our muscles against gravity. When we release the extra muscular effort, it results in a lot of liberated energy. It is easy to say that maintaining an intrinsic equilibrium is a source of energy. In reality, it is only freeing up the energy that you had already been using. Yoga is a way to release stored energy in the axial skeleton by removing the inefficient muscular effort that is obstructing you. It requires a balance of will and a surrender of unnecessary effort to attain the intrinsic equilibrium that is possible through yoga.

Chapter 4: Dhyana: The Meditative Approach to Yoga

As mentioned before, dhyana is a Sanskrit word that means absorption. At its heart, it is the art of reflection, observation and self-study. Through dhyana, you can connect to the divine and develop a profound state of contemplation. It is a way of observing the physical and mental processes of the body.

When the powers of your heart and intellect are blended in harmony, you are using dhyana. All of your creativity proceeds from this state. In many ways, dhyana is like a very deep sleep. While the serenity of sleep normally comes from unconsciously losing your identity and individuality while you rest, someone in a state of meditation brings that serenity along with them while remaining mentally alert. They witness all of the thoughts that arrive and achieve a state of total absorption. In this meditative state, the practitioner can experience illumination.

Dhyana is basically the complete integration of you, the act of contemplation and the object that you are contemplating. With practice, the distinction between yourself and everything else can disappear. You become vibrant, poised and mentally alert in a state that is free from negative emotions like desire or greed. At this point, you can experience the true self and the reflection of the soul.

In normal life, you may experience many contradictions. Your thoughts may not represent your actions or values. You may feel bewildered by the contradictions of life like joy and sorrow, pain and pleasure, conflict and peace. While you may try to find a place of stability that is free from pain and sorrow, it is rare to find a way to do this in your normal existence.

In dhyana, we learn through our meditation that it is possible to reach our inner light and understand the true nature of the world. Following the eight stages of yoga, one can gain insight into life's problems and their solution. As a result, you can strengthen your spirit and work toward the path of liberation.

An untrained mind always wants to flee aimlessly in every direction. In meditation, your mind is taught to move from imperfect knowledge to perfection through will-power and focus. At times, you will experience a harmonious interplay between your thoughts, speech and actions. Your stilled mind becomes like an oil lamp in a windless forest that shines brightly into the night.

There are so many potentials that lie dormant within the heart of man. It is as if the human mind is a fallow field that is lying dormant without crops. A wise man fertilizes, waters and plants the land for a harvest in the future. If you can nourish your fallow mind, you can be like the wise farmer and enjoy the wisdom, clarity and joy that can come from meditation.

The inward journey of meditation is something that takes years of practice, study and discipline. Monks spend decades cultivating their awareness through meditation, so do not expect it to happen overnight. It takes time to expand your consciousness, and meditation must be done on a daily basis.

The Power of Absorption and the Effects of Meditation

Dhyana is best described as a subjective experience of an objective state. This state of mind is difficult to describe in words because it is specific to each person. When meditation is used, the searching ends as the goal and the soul become one. In this moment, the sweet nectar of the infinite can be tasted. With practice, you can become one with the universal soul.

Meditation is a way of finding fulfillment and achieving nirvana. Regardless of your faith, you can achieve exceptional benefits from meditating. This practice has been shown to boost happiness and concentration. In clinical studies, Buddhist monks were given MRIs while meditating. The results were off the charts—quite literally too high to quantify. While all they were doing was meditating, the monks' minds showed happiness levels that had never been seen before by scientists.

Beyond the mental and spiritual benefits, meditation offers a way to lower your blood pressure and improve your cardiovascular health. The many parts of your body are all intricately linked, so the improvement of one organ or the reduction of one hormone can drastically affect another.

In the case of meditation, the focus and relaxation induced help to lower cortisol levels. Known as the stress hormone, cortisol can cause damage to your heart and veins if it continues unchecked. Unfortunately for modern man, the current world is a continued source of stress. You no longer experience stress on the rare occasion that you run from a prehistoric tiger. Instead, your work, traffic, cars driving by, loud music, family life, financial stress and other worries can cause your cortisol levels to rise. When you meditate, you reduce your cortisol levels and increase your overall physical health.

There are essentially two ways to find happiness in life. The first technique is based on external factors like buying prettier clothes, getting a more luxurious house or obtaining a better job. The second option is through mental development that brings about inner happiness.

While many people choose the first option, it is not the most effective way to long-term happiness. In one study, researchers looked at the happiness levels of people who recently won the lottery and individuals who suddenly became paraplegics. At the initial survey, the group that won the lottery was much happier than the group that went from able-bodied to paraplegic. One year later, both groups had similar happiness levels.

Over time, both groups adjusted to their new state of life. Their minds returned to their normal, stable state of happiness. The people who were happy before were still happy afterward no matter what happened to them. Meanwhile, the people who had negative outlooks remained unhappy a year later whether they lost a limb or won the lottery. This study tells us that it is the internal state of happiness that matters. Unless you found a way to win the lottery or have only positive moments occur every day for the rest of your life, any external source of happiness will not last.

In the West, we think of yoga as a physical process that allows us to become fit and healthy. While it will do this, the entire yogic practice and eight stages can go beyond physical fitness. When you practice all eight stages of yoga, you have a chance at developing internal, lasting happiness.

Traditional yogic texts and Buddhism teach us that we are all born into a state of suffering.

Sickness, hunger, pain and suffering of all types are something that everyone must deal with. At the end of life, we must all die and leave our current form. Yoga and meditation are the traditional ways to break free from the cycle of suffering and experience liberation from the pain. Negative things can happen to you, but what matters is how your mind perceives them and reacts.

Breaking Down the Analytical Brain

During meditation, the mind returns to its origin to find a spiritual haven. In this state, the yogi is able to break down the polarity that exists between the analytical dominant consciousness of the front half of the brain and the subconsciousness of the back half of the brain. When this happens, the yogi is able to see the underlying reality that exists around him.

Normally, the brain is stimulated by external factors that disturb the consciousness. When the mind is at peace, automatic physical functions like the heart beat, intestinal contractions and breathing are slowed. The meditative mind and matter are fused together in a way that burns out all distracting thoughts. At this point, you reach your creative, attentive and dynamic center. You are able to achieve an inexhaustible reserve of energy and focus on bettering yourself.

When you have practiced meditation for a long time, you are able to reach a new dimension where all of your senses become clear. It is like all of the waves of a lake dying down and still water emerging to hold a mirror up to yourself. Your soul remains awake, but your senses are now under control. In this state, you can enjoy exceptional knowledge, freedom, illumination and truth.

Using Mantras in Meditation

While every meditation practice varies, mantra meditation is commonly used by beginners. This type of meditation is ideal for keeping your mind from wandering as you meditate. In the beginning, say the mantra aloud. As you become better at focusing your mind, you can begin to say the mantra mentally. In Sanskrit, mantra meditation is known as sagarbha dhyana. Silent meditation without a mantra is often referred to as agarbha dhyana.

Before you truly begin your meditation practice, you just learn to differentiate between the emptiness and peace of meditation and the illumination of the spirit. Dhyana consists of three categories: sattvic, tamasic and rajasic. It is best to maintain a sattvic meditation practice because it will keep you on the path of truth and illumination.

Your body is referred to as the city of Brahma. Within your "city", there are nine gates: the reproductive organs, mouth, anus, eyes, nostrils and ears. All of these gates are supposed to be closed during meditation. When the gates are closed and your chakras are in harmony, your mind is able to be at peace.

During meditation, the brain must be balanced correctly above the spine. If there is any unevenness in your spine and neck, it will disturb the tranquility of your meditation. When the left and right hemispheres of the brain are balanced correctly, it allows your mind to center itself and thinking activity in your mind comes to a stop. This is similar to the way that ceasing the movement of a limb causes it to become passive. When the flow of energy to the brain is reduced, you can focus on the heart and become just a passive observer in the brain.

You can use any mantra that suits your current life, needs or problems. While "om" is a traditional mantra, Sanskrit words like "ananda" (bliss) are also commonly used. If using Sanskrit and mentally translating the mantra is difficult for you, you can also pick a mantra in your native language that suits you. Mantras can be repeated for any amount of time, or you can use mala beads to keep track of your repetitions.

Attaining the Best Posture for Meditation

To achieve physical and mental harmony during meditation, you must be able to sit properly. While some types of meditation do not require you to sit, it is the ideal position. Start by raising the front and back halves of your body evenly. Focus on keeping your spine straight and your chest lifted upward. This position causes your breathing to slow down and encourages activity in the brain to lessen.

As you begin to meditate, your goal is to keep your body and mind alert with a razor-sharp awareness. At the same time, your brain should passive and sensitive. If you allow your body to collapse, it will cause mental dullness and distract your mind.

During meditation, your head should be parallel to the ceiling. It should not be tilted in any way. According to tradition, a head that is facing downward indicates a tamasic mind that is brooding on the past. When your head is facing too far upward, it shows that your mind is rajasic as you imagine the future. A steady head shows that you are present in the moment with a sattvic state of mind.

Especially in the beginning, you should close your eyes and look inward. Shut your eyes to any noises and listen to the inward sound of yourself. By closing your eyes and ears, you can direct your focus upon the meditation instead of on the outward world.

Ideally, you do not want to sit for meditation immediately after pranayama or asanas. Only experienced meditators are able to do pranayama and dhyana together. Your best option is to meditate at a time when your body and mind are refreshed. If you can still be alert, before bedtime could also be an option since your mind is at a state of peace.

Chapter 5: Asanas for Daily Practice: Sun Salutations to Greet the Day

While there are hundreds and hundreds of asanas that you can do every day, one of the best ways to start your day is with the Sun Salutation set (surya namaskar). The postures help to calm your mind while keeping your body fit and healthy. It is best to do Sun Salutations in the early morning before you have eaten. Each Sun Salutation is done with a set of 12 yoga poses. If you want to modify the poses or add in new ones, you will want to do two rounds so that your muscles do not become unbalanced. This is because the first round is done with moving the left leg, while the second round is done by moving the right leg.

Depending on your physical health, you may want to make modifications to these yoga poses.

Your body knows what is best for you, so listen to it. With regular practice, Sun Salutations can help to improve your muscular strength and concentration. Traditionally, Sun Salutations were done as an expression of gratitude to the sun for supporting life on our planet. When you finish both rounds of the Sun Salutations, relax in corpse pose until you are fully ready to start your day.

Mountain Pose (Tadasana)

In this pose, you will want to stand at the edge of your mat with your feet together. Balance your weight so that your weight is equally spread out. Relax your shoulders and let your chest expand. Bring the palms of your hand together at your heart and imagine a sun shining brightly from your heart. As you inhale, you are causing the sun to shine brighter. Give thanks for the life-giving energy provided by the sun and the life force (prana) that flows through all living beings.

This pose receives its name because "tada" means mountain. While your crown reaches toward the heavens, your feet remain firmly rooted in the ground like a mountain. This pose is especially good for regaining strength in your feet. In ancient man, the feet were strengthened by running, walking and standing barefoot. Since humans now wear shoes all the time, the feet can develop problems like plantar fasciitis and heel spurs. Standing postures like tadasana help to restore the natural adaptability and vitality of the feet.

Upward Salute (Urdhva Hastasana)

As you inhale, turn your palms so that they face outward. Bring your arms over your head as you sweep upward. Allow your spine to gently bend backwards to open up your chest and lift the heart. This pose is symbolic for opening yourself to life. Focus your gaze upward as you relax your forehead and keep your facial expression soft. "Urdhva" means upward, and "hasta" means hands. Thus, this pose means that your hands turn upwards.

Standing Forward Bend (Uttanasana)

As you breathe out, bend forward from your waist and allow your spine to stay erect. Bring your hands down to the floor beside each of your foot. If you cannot touch the floor without bending your knees, it is fine to modify this pose by allowing your knees to bend slightly. Each day, try to straighten your knees a little more.

While "ut" means intense, "tan" means to stretch. Because of this, you can think of the standing forward bend as an intense stretch. This exercise helps to passively lengthen the spinal muscles while maintaining your knee extension. With practice, it can help to strengthen muscles like the adductor magnus, the hamstrings, the gluteus medius, the gluteus minimus and the gastrocnemius. Ideally, gravity should do most of the work when it comes to deepening your pose.

Half Standing Forward Bend (Ardha Uttanasana)

Inhale deeply as you lift your gaze. This causes your chest and chin to lift along with the gaze. While your legs stay rooted strongly in the ground, reach down toward your shins. Press your hands into the shins to help straighten out your spine and lift your heart. Let your breath fill you up as you enjoy this moment. Your breath should always guide your movement as you focus on each inhale and exhale. Likewise, your mental gaze should follow the direction of the movement.

Four-Limbed Staff Pose (Chaturanga Dandasana)

Exhale as you step back into plank pose. As you do this, shift your weight toward the front as you bend your arms. Allow your body to be lowered until your upper arms are next to your side ribs and parallel to the ground. Do not allow your hips or core to sink. This pose allows you to surrender your ego and offer your heart as you prostrate yourself on the ground. If you need to modify the pose, lower your knees to the ground.

"Chatur" means four, and "anga" means limb. Meanwhile, "danda" means staff, which gives the pose the name of the four-limbed staff. This pose helps to strengthen the quadriceps, pectoralis major, gluteus maximus, triceps and oblique muscles. As you improve in this pose, you will develop better strength that lets you breathe smoothly for a longer period of time.

Upward-Facing Dog Pose (Urdhva Mukha Svanasana)

As you inhale, press backward onto your toes so that you are on the tops of your feet. At the same time, press your hands down as you draw your shoulders backward. This helps to widen your chest while letting your inhalation naturally fill your lungs. Make sure that you keep your legs and feet activated in the pose. Your gaze should be lifted to just past the top of your nose. If you find this pose difficult, you can do cobra pose (bhujangasana) instead.

This pose takes its name from the words "urdhva" (rising), "mukha" (face) and "shvana" (dog). It activates the muscles of the hamstrings, diaphragm, spinal extensors, triceps and psoas major. When you hold the pose for several breaths, it allows you to deepen the extension of your thoracic spine. Each exhale will help to stabilize your cervical and lumbar curves.

Downward-Facing Dog Pose (Adho Mukha Svanasana)

As you exhale, tuck your toes under your body and use your core strength to bring your hips upward. Create a straight line that runs through your wrists, shoulders, hips and spine. If you need to modify the pose, you can place your feet farther apart or lift your heels from the ground. Allow the back of your neck to relax and stay in the pose for at least five breaths. While the pose requires strength, it should not strain you. If you are overwhelmed, drop down into child's pose for the remainder of your breaths.

This pose comes from the names "adho" (downward), "mukha" (face) and "shvana"(dog). Downward-facing dog is an excellent pose to see how the arms and legs affect the spine. It activates the muscles in the back, bottom and back legs. Keep your core activated in the pose, and each inhale will cause your thoracic structures to mobilize.

Feet to Hands

This pose allows you to transition from downward-facing dog to half standing forward band. After five exhales, step or jump your feet forward so that they meet your hands.

Half Standing Forward Bend (Ardha Uttanasana)

As you inhale, lift your chin and allow your chest and gaze to follow. Straighten out your spine. You can use your hands on your thighs to help straighten your spine out as you hold the pose. "Ardha" means half, and "ut" means intense. "Tan" is the Sanskrit word for stretch. Because of this, ardha uttanasa means half of an intense stretch.

Standing Forward Bend (Uttanasana)

Return to standing forward bend by exhaling and allowing yourself to fold completely. Let your back soften as you curl downward. If you cannot keep your hands flat on the ground, place them on the top of your feet or legs as gravity works to pull yourself downward.

Upward Salute (Urdhva Hastasana)

As you reach the end of the Sun Salutations, inhale and allow your body to rise fully. Straighten out the spine, look up and return to upward salute.

Mountain Pose (Tadasana)

Exhale and bring yourself back to mountain pose. Pause for a moment as you allow your chest and heart to open up. From this point, you could continue to do other poses, end your yoga practice for the day, meditate or relax in corpse pose.

Remember to Follow Your Breath

To test the full experience of the Sun Salutations (surya namaskar), remember to let your breath lead the movement. Each inhale and exhale should bring you to the next pose naturally, so do not force this to happen. You are following the source of your prana by following the breath and experiencing the heart of yoga. Since this sequence is intended as a gesture of gratitude for the sun, you can allow your mind to thank the elements and the sun for allowing life to happen.

For a variation of this approach, you can add a mantra into your movements. This can activate the spiritual nature of the poses, and it allows you to finish feeling more relaxed. While you can use basic mantras like "om", you can also try the Vedic mantra, the Gayatri mantra or one of your own choosing.

The Meanings Behind Popular Asanas

The Tree (Vrikshasana)

Of the many asanas, the tree pose has remained one of my favorites. In this pose, you must have a deeply rooted stance and balance, or you will end up falling over. It is amazing how much your mental attitude, focus and worries from life influence your ability to do the tree pose. When you are focused on stress from work, it seems impossible to stay balanced.

In this pose, one knee is brought out to the side in a standing position. This opens up the pelvis as the raised foot balances on your upper thigh. Once you have brought your leg up, you bring your arms above your head or lower them into prayer position. The pose takes its name from the tree because, like a tree, its stability depends on your base. In ancient China, trees were thought to be the souls of the gods and were sacred.

Spinal Twist (Ardha Matsyendrasana)

"Ardha" means half, and "Matsyendra" is the name of a sage who once spread the teachings of yoga. In this particular pose, the right leg is placed on the floor and bent so that the foot is on the outside of your left buttock. The left leg is bent and left upright so that it is on the outside of your right thigh. Meanwhile, your body twists to the left as the right arm passes around the bent knee until it clasps your left hand behind the back. Your head turns to the left to look behind.

Twisting the spine is symbolic for your mental ability to bend and see new perspectives. It forces you to adopt a new perspective and is ideal for someone who is set on achieving a spiritual goal.

Camel (Ustrasana)

Like most yoga poses, this one is aptly named: "ustra" means camel in Sanskrit. To do this pose, start by kneeling on the floor with your thighs and feet together. Point your toes backward away from you. To prepare yourself for the pose and prevent injuries, start by resting your palms on your hips. Curve the spine slightly as you hold for several breaths. Uncurve your spine again. Now, do the actual pose. Return to the curved spine position and place your palms over your heels as you exhale. Throw back your head and push the spine towards your thighs. You should remain in this position for at least one minute.

This asana is ideal for anyone who suffers from drooping shoulders or a hunched back. Since it stretches the entire spine, it is ideal for building strength in the spine, but it is not advisable for someone with a back injury. It is a useful pose for the elderly since it helps to prevent the degradation of the spine during aging.

King of the Dancers (Natarjasana)

Named after Siva, Lord of the Dance, this pose comes from the words "nata" (dancer) and "raja" (king). In mythology, Siva was the god of mystical stillness, death and the dance. He lived in the Himalayas and created over a hundred dances. In one terrible dance known as the tandava, Siva, became infuriated at his father-in-law for killing his spouse. He surrounded his attendants as he beat a wild rhythm and destroyed the father-in-law. In honor of him, the vigorous dancer pose was made.

To do this pose, you have to start in a standing position. Stretch out your left arm parallel to the floor. Bending the right knee, use your right arm to pull the right foot. Simultaneously try to stretch your right arm behind your head as you rotate the right elbow. Your right thigh will end up being parallel to the floor. If you can, you can try to deepen this pose. When you are done, make sure to do the pose again on the other side as well.

This pose is ideal for teaching balance and pose. At the same time, it helps to strengthen the leg muscles and allows the chest to expand completely. All of the vertebrae in your spine benefit when you do this pose correctly.

Cobra (Bhujangasana)

Cobra comes from the word, "bhujanga", which means serpent. This backward-bending pose helps to strengthen your serratus anterior, triceps, hamstrings and gluteus maximus muscles. Start the pose by lying flat on the ground with your face pointing downward. Extend your legs behind you with your feet kept together. Your toes should be pointing backward as your knees remain tightly together. Rest the palms of your hands near your pelvis.

When you inhale, press your palms into the ground as you pull your trunk up. Take two breaths. Next, inhale and lift your body from the trunk until your pelvis is in contact with the floor. Remain in this position with most of your weight focused on your legs and hands. Maintain the pose for about 20 seconds.

When done correctly, this posture can help heal an injured spine and strengthen the spinal discs. It is important to do the pose under the supervision of a teacher if you have spinal problems because cobra can worsen a spinal condition if you do it incorrectly.

Bridge (Setu Bandhasana)

This pose is called bridge in English because "setu" means bridge and "bandha" means lock. As a result, you are locking your body into a bridge. With this pose, you can strengthen your abdominal muscles, your gluteus maximus, the hamstrings and your quadriceps.

To do the bridge pose, lie flat with your back on the floor. Take several deep breaths. Bend your knees and bring your heels toward your bottom. As you lift your stomach and chest upward, place your arms underneath your spine for added support. There are many modifications of this pose, so you could try it with your hands above your head pressing into the ground. Advanced yogis will even do the bridge with only their feet and head on the ground!

Like many yoga poses, this asana is ideal for strengthening the spine. In addition to strengthening all parts of the spine, it helps to tone the neck and the extensor muscles of the back. When done properly, the hips are contracted and the spine is well-supported. This pose can stimulate the adrenal, pituitary, thyroid and pineal glands.

Warrior I (Virabhadrasana I)

This pose is named after a fierce warrior from mythology and is often included in sets of Sun

Salutations. In mythology, Daksa celebrated a sacrifice, but did not invite his daughter or her husband, Siva, who was the chief of the gods. His daughter was completely humiliated and threw herself on a fire to die. Her husband, Siva, heard the news and became enraged. Provoked, he called on his best warrior, Virabhadra, to lead Siva's army and destroy the sacrifice. Led by Virabhadra, the army appeared at Daksa's sacrifice and beheaded him. In grief for his wife, Siva then left to meditate.

To do this pose, start in tadasana. Raise both of your arms above your head and stretch toward the sky. With a deep inhalation, take a step forward with your back foot almost perpendicular to your front foot. Bend your front knee, but make sure that it does not overshadow your ankle. Instead, the front knee should be in line with the front heel. Stretch your back leg outward and let it tighten. Hold the pose for 20 seconds before repeating it on the other side. When you are done, return to tadasana.

Warrior I is an excellent pose for expanding your chest and improves breathing. While it works to tone the muscles in the knees and ankles, Warrior I also works to relieve any stiffness in the shoulders and back. It can remove stiffness in the neck and reduce the fat that gathers around your hips.

Warrior II (Virabhadrasana II)

From tadasana, take a deep inhale and then jump one of your legs forward several feet. Raise your arms sideways so that your arms are parallel to your legs. The palms should be facing down. Next, turn your back foot sideways about 90 degrees. Like Warrior I, your front knee should be bent and your back leg should be straight. Continue to stretch your hands sideways as you gaze toward the front hand. Remain in this pose for 20 seconds before repeating it for the other side.

When you do this pose regularly, it helps you to develop shapely, athletic legs. If you have cramps in your thighs or calves, Warrior II can help to relieve them. Meanwhile, it also works to strengthen your abdominal muscles. Standing poses are ideal for beginners to use to prepare themselves for advanced poses later on.

Warrior III (Virabhadrasana III)

In this modification of the basic Warrior I pose, you will again start in tadasana. With a deep inhalation, step forward with one leg so that the front leg is bent at the knee and the back leg is straight. Exhale and bend the top of your body forward until your chest rests on your front thigh. Keep your palms together and maintain your arms as straight as possible.

At this point, you can hold the pose for 20 seconds before returning to tadasana or you can deepen the pose. If you want to deepen the pose, exhale and lift your back leg from the ground. Swing your body forward slightly as you straighten out your leg so that it is parallel to the floor. Hold your leg in the air like this for 20 to 30 seconds as you breathe deeply. Your bottom leg should be straight and perpendicular to the floor. With an exhale, return to Warrior I or tadasana before doing the other side.

Warrior III requires an exceptional level of balance. When you do this pose, it makes your abdominal muscles contract and strengthen. As the abdominal muscles contract, it helps to tone your internal organs. Meanwhile, the pose also works to strengthen your legs. This pose is ideal for improving your natural posture and bearing. By improving your posture, your mental state is affected and you are able to enjoy a greater peace of mind and mental agility.

Child's Pose (Balasana)

In Sanskrit, "bala" means young or childish. This pose uses gravity to naturally deepen the position. With practice, child's pose can improve your diaphragm, spine, hamstrings and calves. Kneeling on the ground, sit with your feet tucked under your body. Lean down so that your forehead touches the ground. Next, bring your arms to your sides so that your palms face toward the ceiling. The goal of this pose is to bring your sitting bones to the heels and your forehead to the floor. As you improve, you will be able to get closer to achieving this goal.

Supported Shoulder Stand (Salamba Sarvangasana)

This pose receives its name from the words "salamba" (with support), "sarva" (all) and "anga" (limbs). To start this pose, lie flat on your back. Keep your legs stretched out with the knees tightened. Put your hands on the sides of your legs with the palms facing down. Take several deep breaths.

As you exhale, bend your knees and move your legs toward your stomach until your thighs press into your stomach. Take two more breaths. Then, raise your hips from the floor as you exhale and place both of your hands behind your back with your elbows bent. Take two breaths. At your next exhale, straighten your legs so that they are perpendicular in the air. If you are experienced, you can remain in this position for five minutes as you breathe evenly. With each exhale, allow your hands to gradually slide down until you can release them completely. If you cannot do it without support, you can use a stool or a wall to prop up your legs.

It would be impossible to underestimate the benefits of the supported shoulder stand. It helps to stimulate the endocrine organs and can help with a wide range of ailments. The blood supply flows down to the head in this pose, which encourages strong circulation and can relieve breathing conditions. Likewise, the gravity works to improve the functioning of the bowels and digestive system. If you have been ill and are only returning to practice, this pose can help to make up for lost vitality.

Corpse Pose (Savasana)

It is only fitting that a book of yoga would finish with the last pose traditionally included in yoga class. Corpse pose (savasana) takes its name because it looks as if you are a corpse. The posture is designed to stimulate a dead body with your figure flat upon the ground, legs slightly apart and arms relaxed on the ground. It is the ideal pose for relaxation and recuperation. Because of this, many yoga teachers use corpse pose as the last pose in class to allow your body and mind time to recuperate before you leave. It is during corpse pose that the benefits of the day are realized.

While lying on the ground may be relaxing, the perfect savasana requires exceptional discipline. It is simple to relax and feel at ease for a few moments, but extremely difficult to maintain for extended periods of time. When you perform savasana correctly, your ribs become like a string of pearls. Each breath causes the string of pearls to move together in harmony. The body, breath and mind move slowly as everything returns to a state of balance.

It is normal in the beginning for your ribs and your breath to have problems relaxing. Through controlled physical and mental discipline, you can achieve a stillness and peace. In the silence, your attention expands and releases as your will submerges with the universe.

Chapter 6: Conclusion: Developing a Lifelong Practice

Western thought and methods can only take you so far in freeing your mind and body. Eastern philosophy and yoga enable you to take the next step on the path to liberation. Your asana practice will help you to live a happier, healthier life. While you may have little time to practice, even 15 minutes a day can go a long way toward improving your outlook on life.

It can take many years of practice before you develop insights into your mind, the Self and your personal spirituality. Even before years have passed, you will immediately start to notice benefits from your practice. From waking up refreshed to enjoying better physical health, there are many immediate benefits to a daily yoga practice.